Things I Want to Say to My Patients But I Can't

Swearing Adult Colouring Books for Nurses

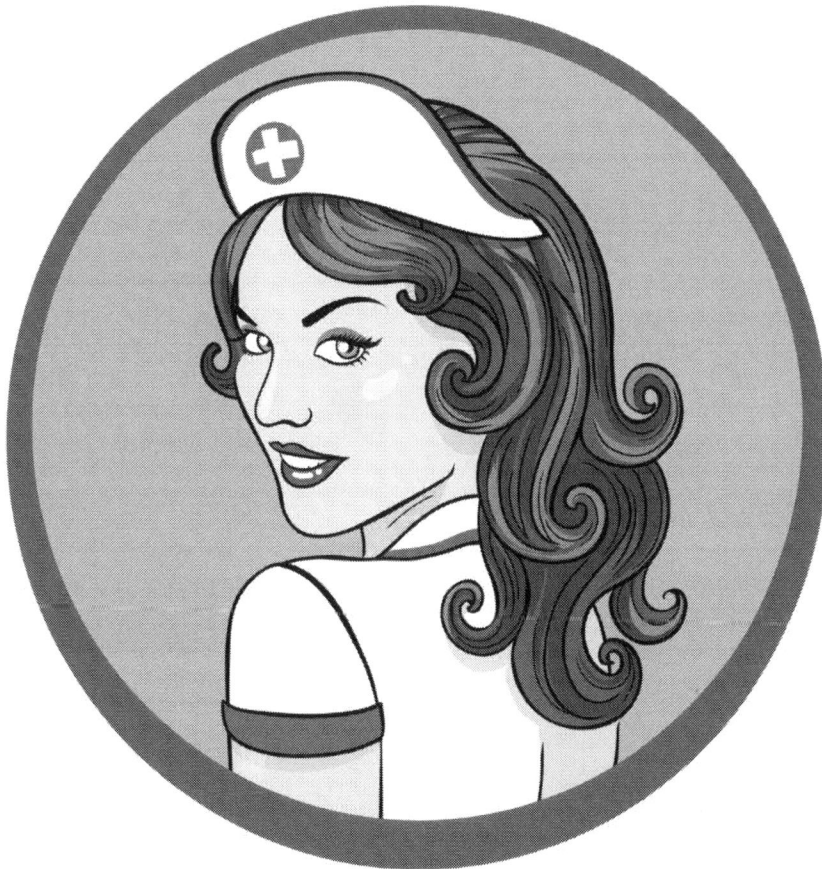

by Shut Up Coloring

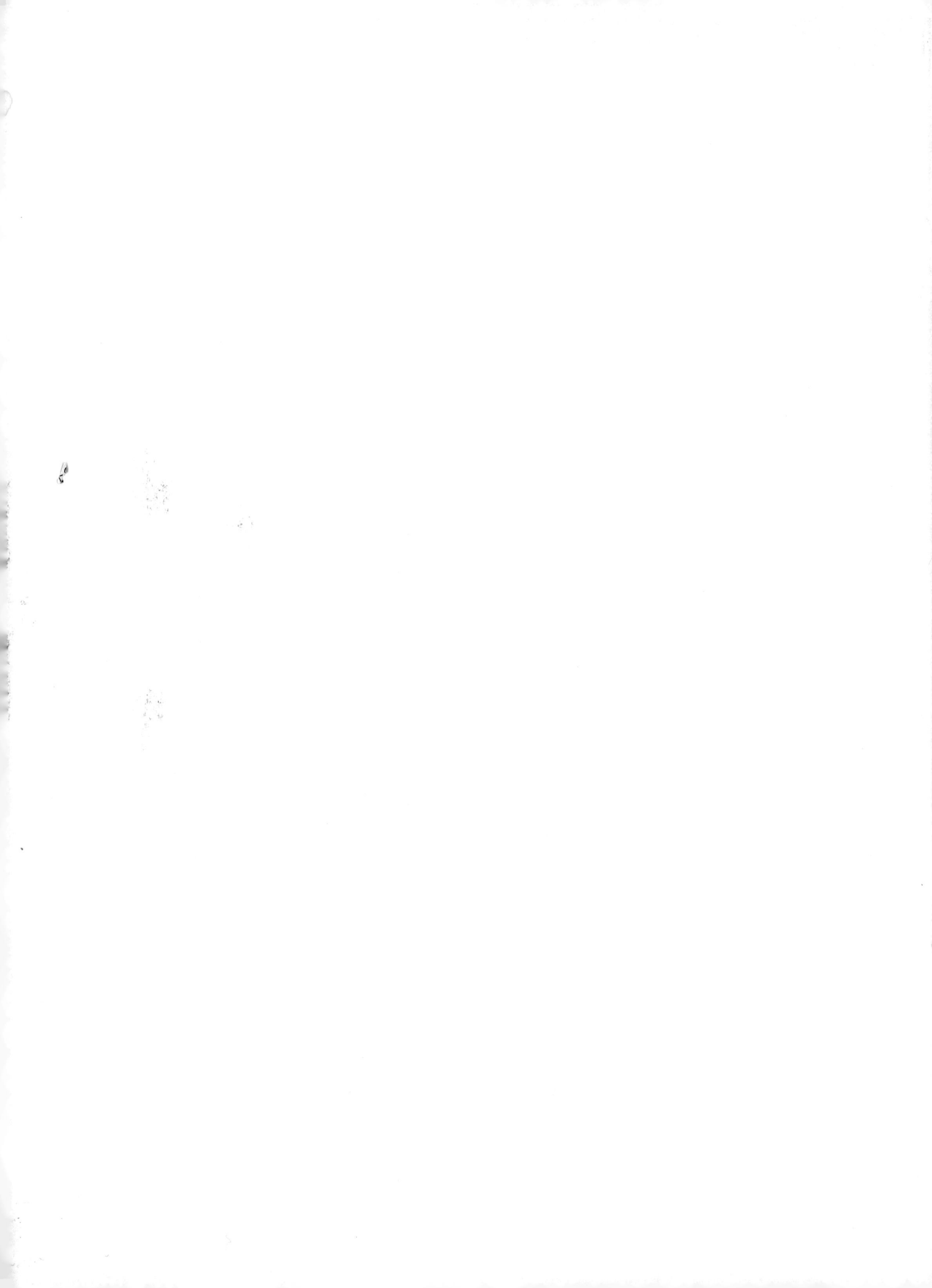

STOP SHITTING THE BED FUCKER

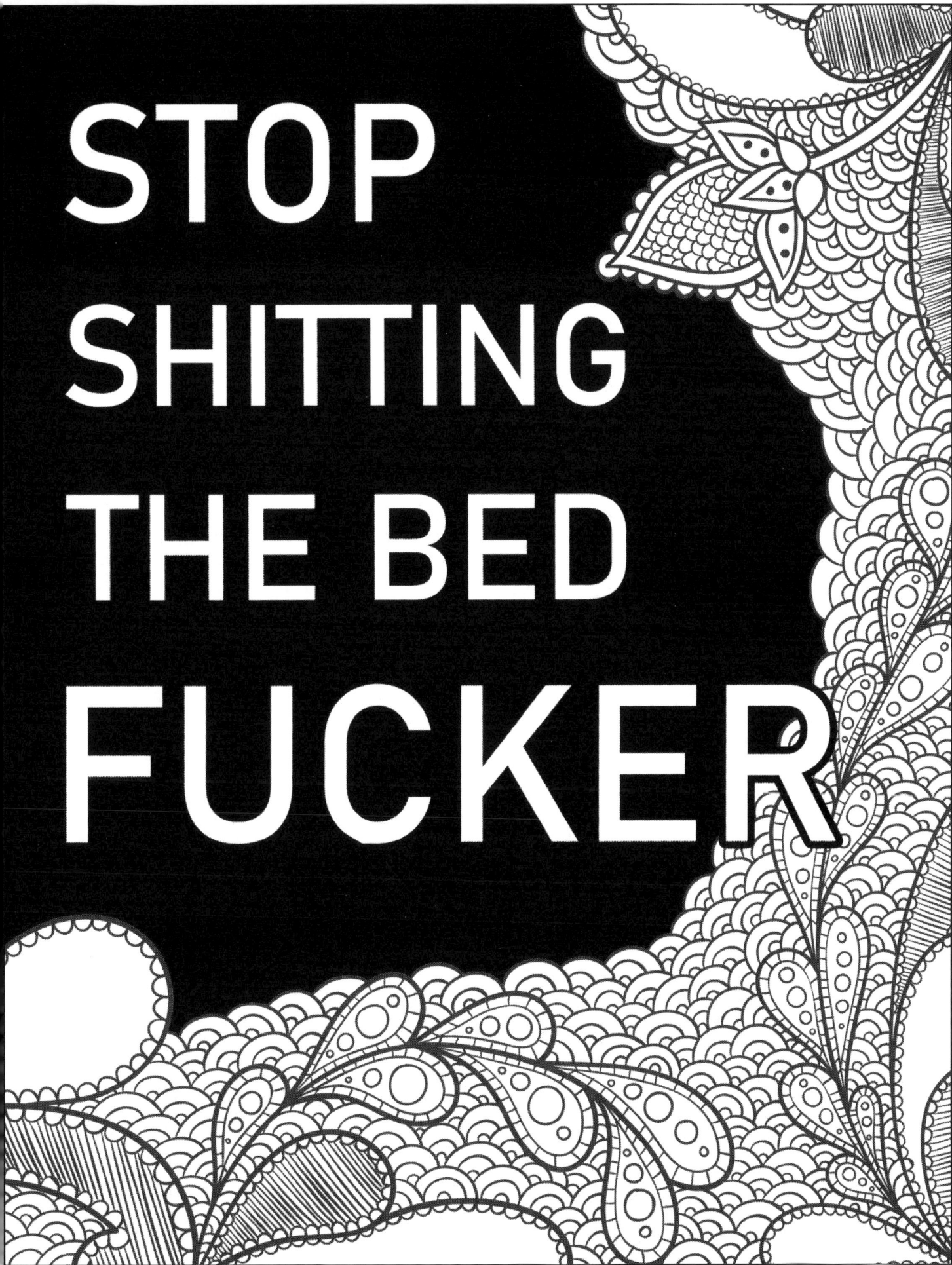

I NEED A MOTHERFUCKING NAP

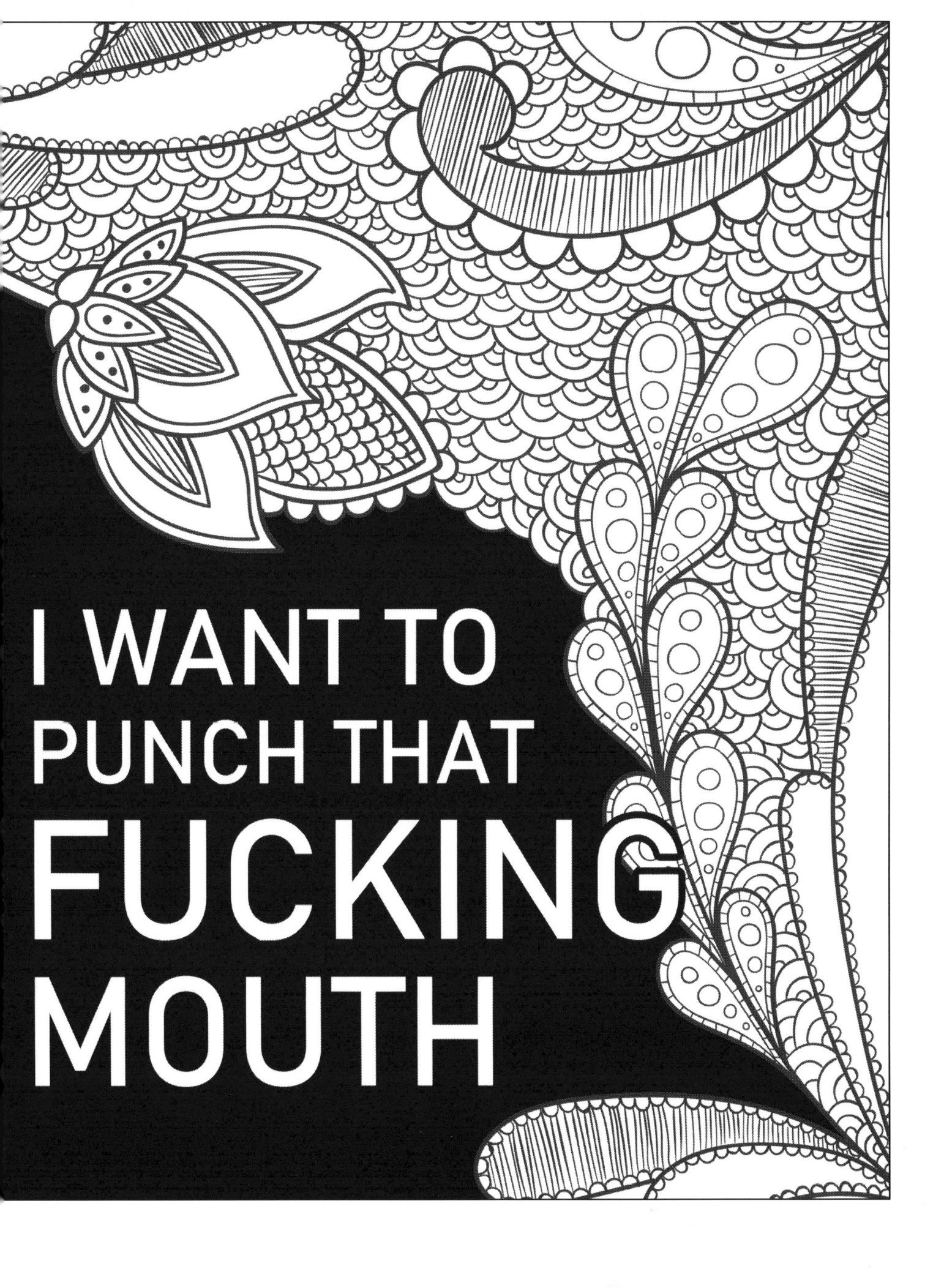

I WANT TO
PUNCH THAT
FUCKING
MOUTH

BE FUCKING NICE TO ME I MAYBE YOUR NURSE SOMEDAY

IT TAKE A BIG HEART

HEART

TO SAVE LIFE OF

DIPSHITS

WAKE UP ASSHOLE

YOUR THUMB IS PAIN
BECAUSE
HITTING THE FUCKING
CALL BUTTON EVERY MINUTE

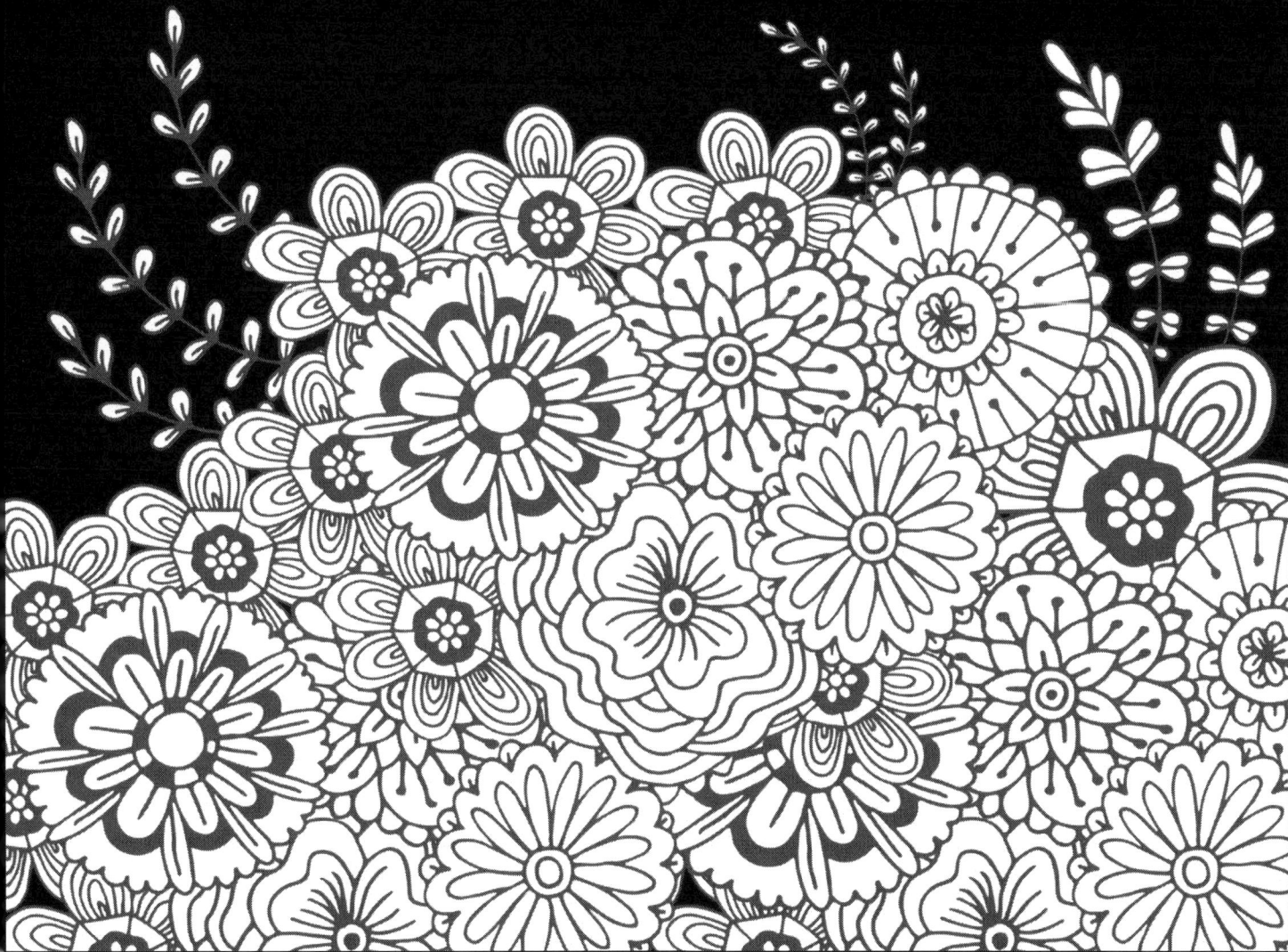

IT TOOK ME 5 MINUTES

TO GET YOUR PILLS

BECAUSE SOME POOR FUCKER

IS DYING

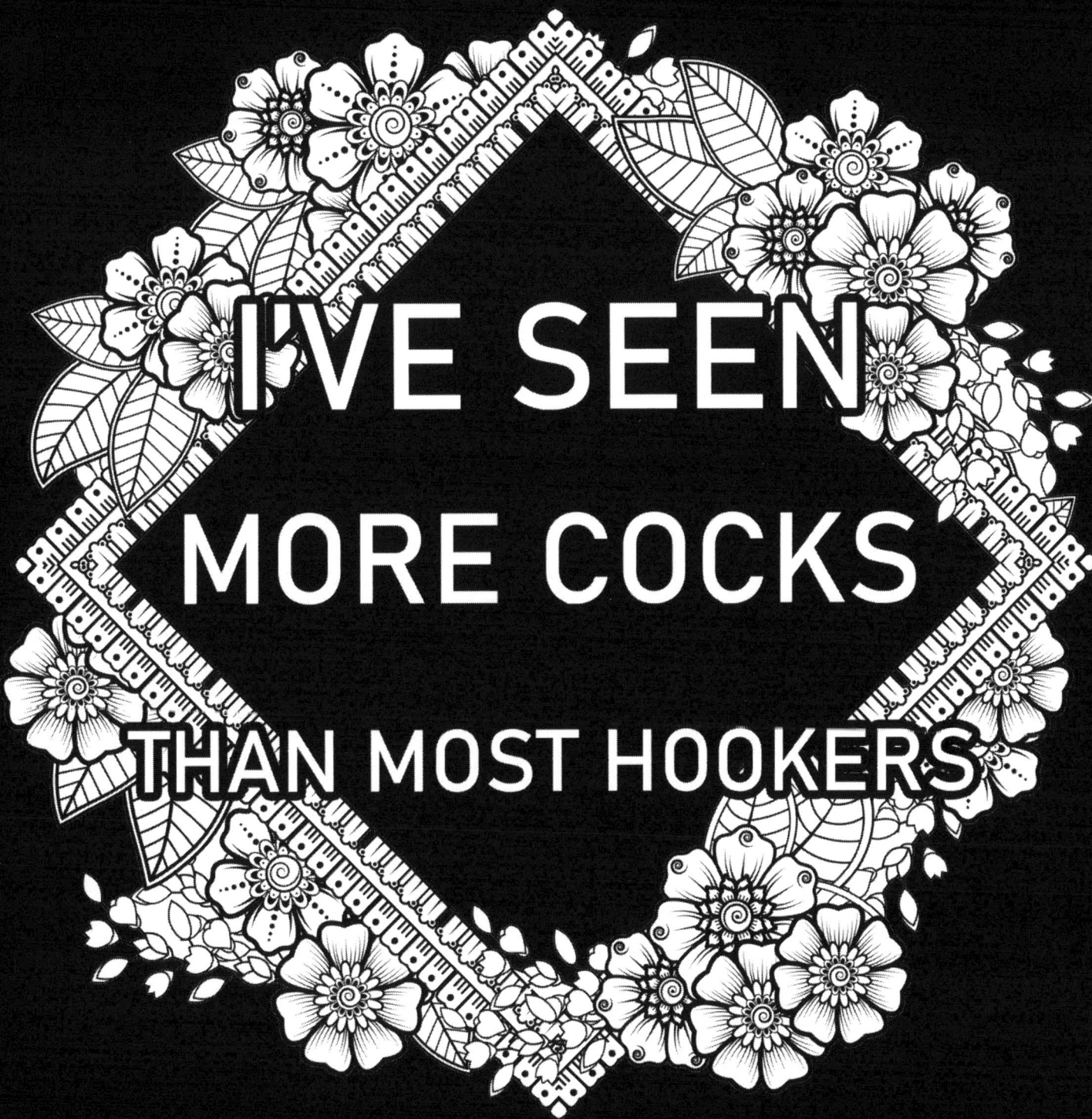

I'VE SEEN MORE COCKS THAN MOST HOOKERS

TRY TO NICE
TO
DICK HEADS
IS THE HARDEST PART
TO BEING NURSE

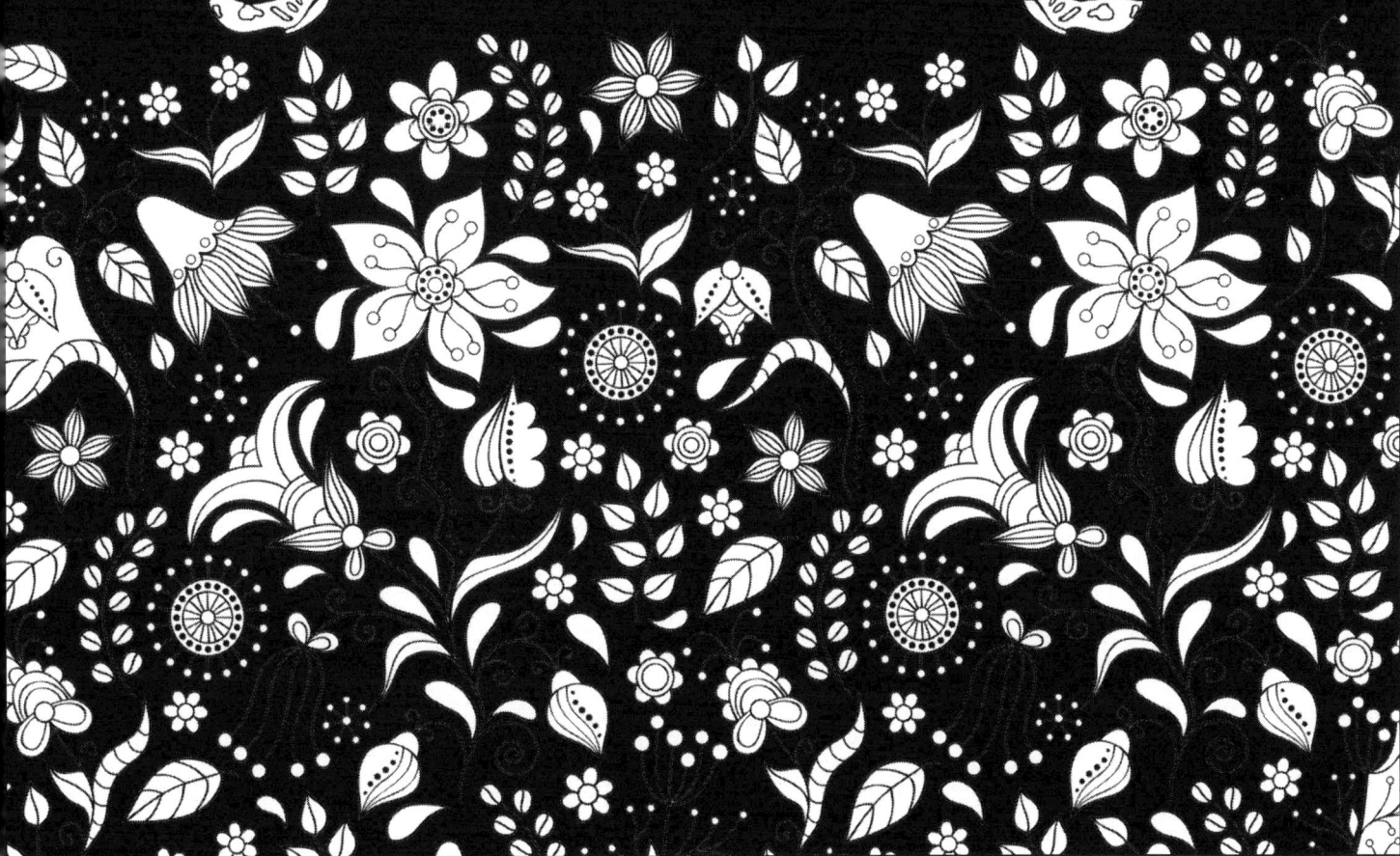

I SEE YOU

HAVE A SEVERE

CASE OF FUCKING

PRETENDINITIS

THE MOST MOVIES THAT I WATCH IS FIFTY SHADE OF SHITS

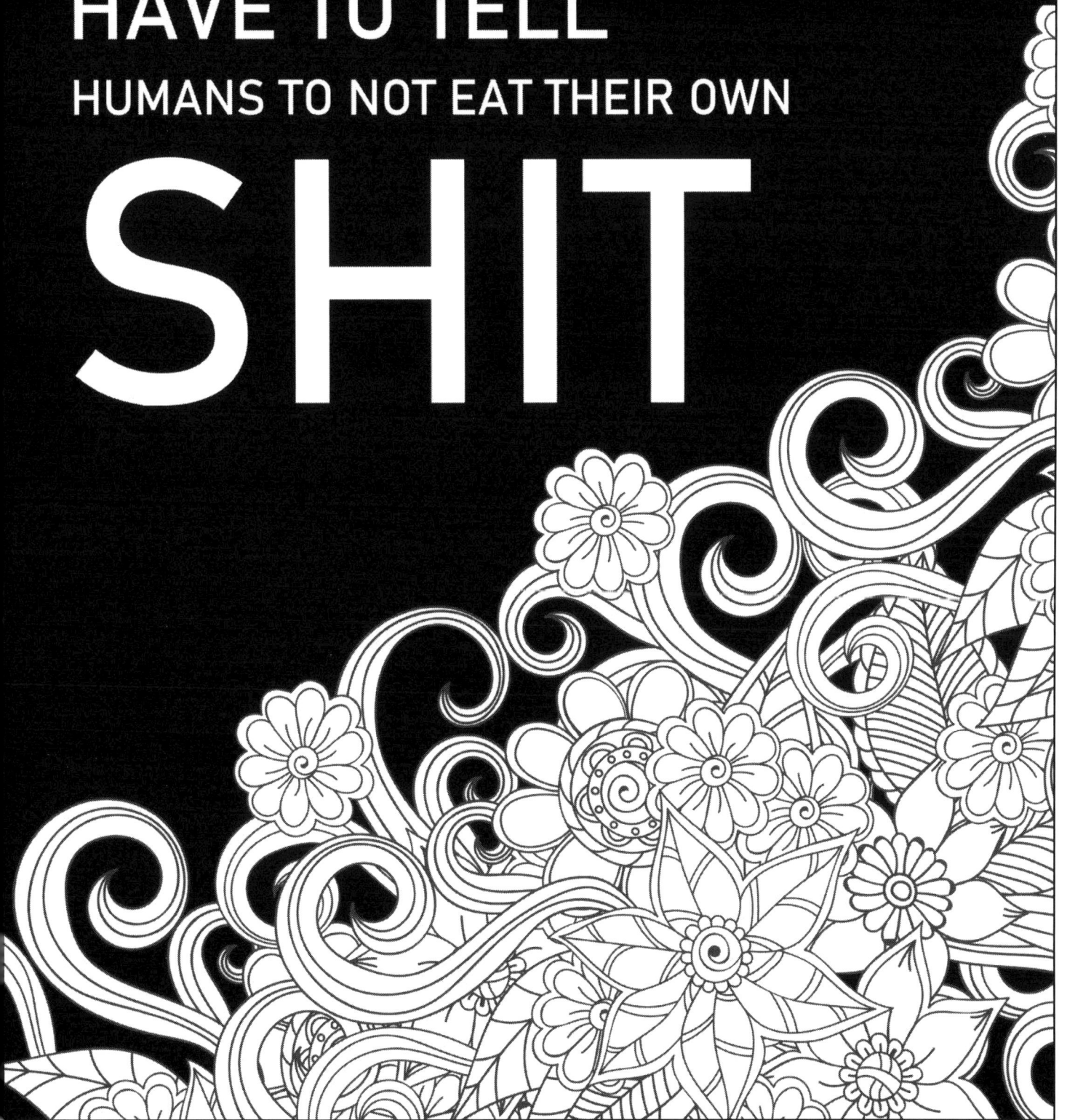

I SHOULDN'T
HAVE TO TELL
HUMANS TO NOT EAT THEIR OWN
SHIT

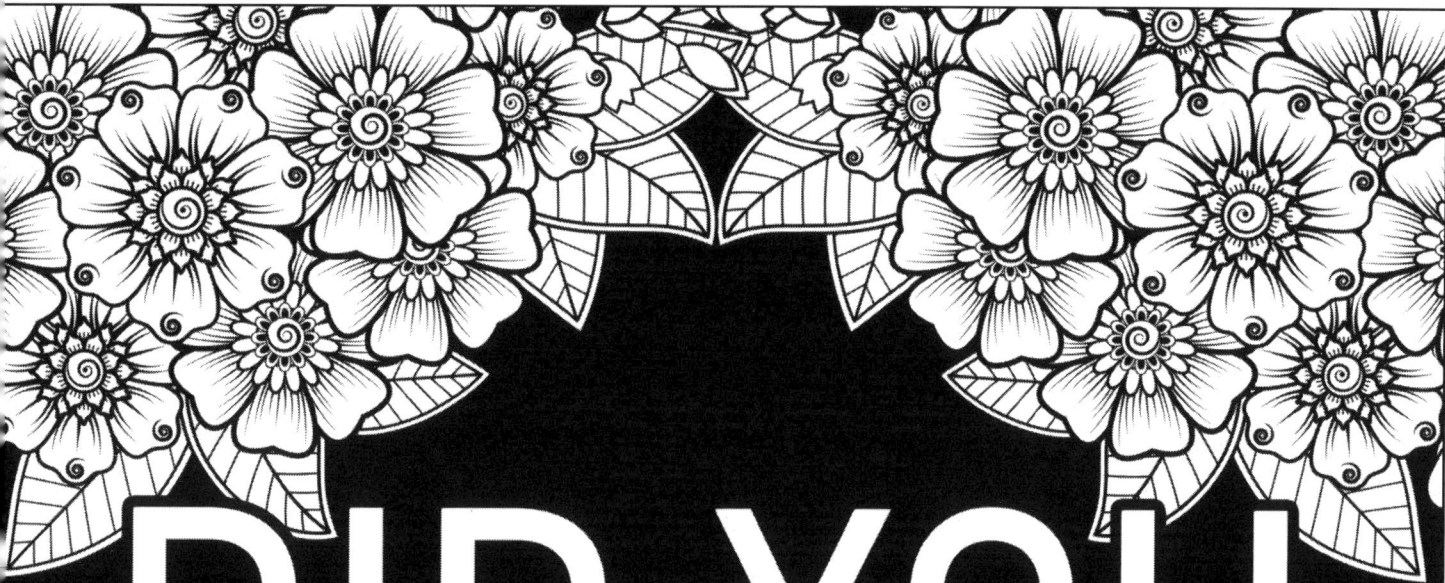

DID YOU JUST SHIT

YOUR PANTS AGAIN?

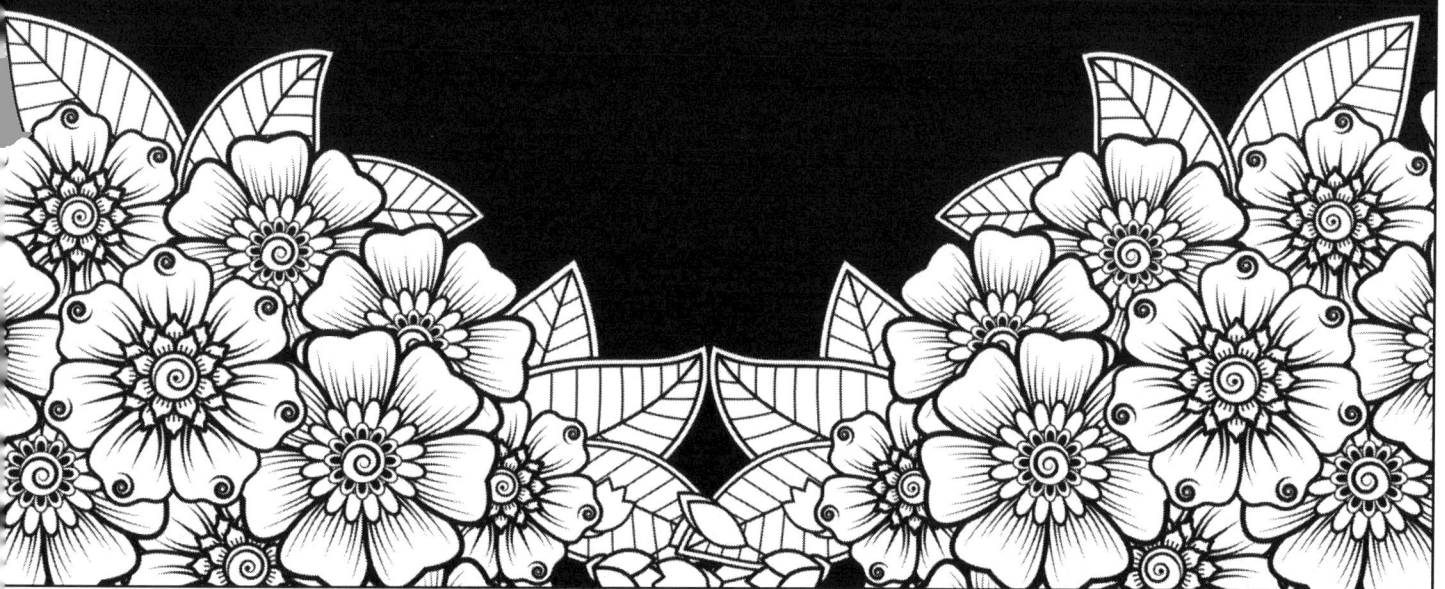

I'VE GOT A GOOD

HEART

BUT THIS FUCKING

MOUTH

I LOVE MY FUCKING PATIENTS

I SEE MORE SHIT THAN PATIENTS

THIS NURSE NEEDS A MOTHER FUCKING NAP

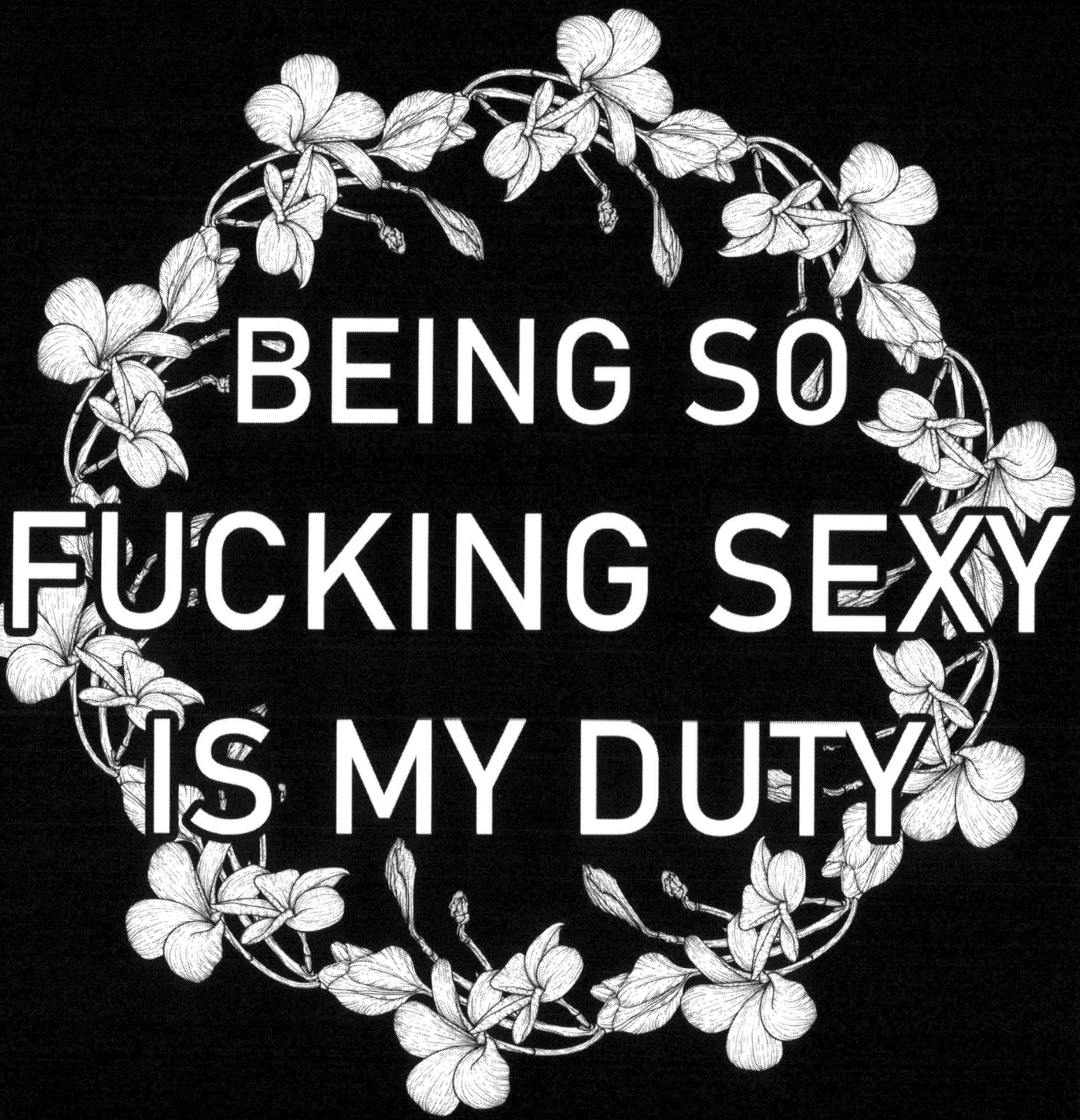

BEING SO FUCKING SEXY IS MY DUTY

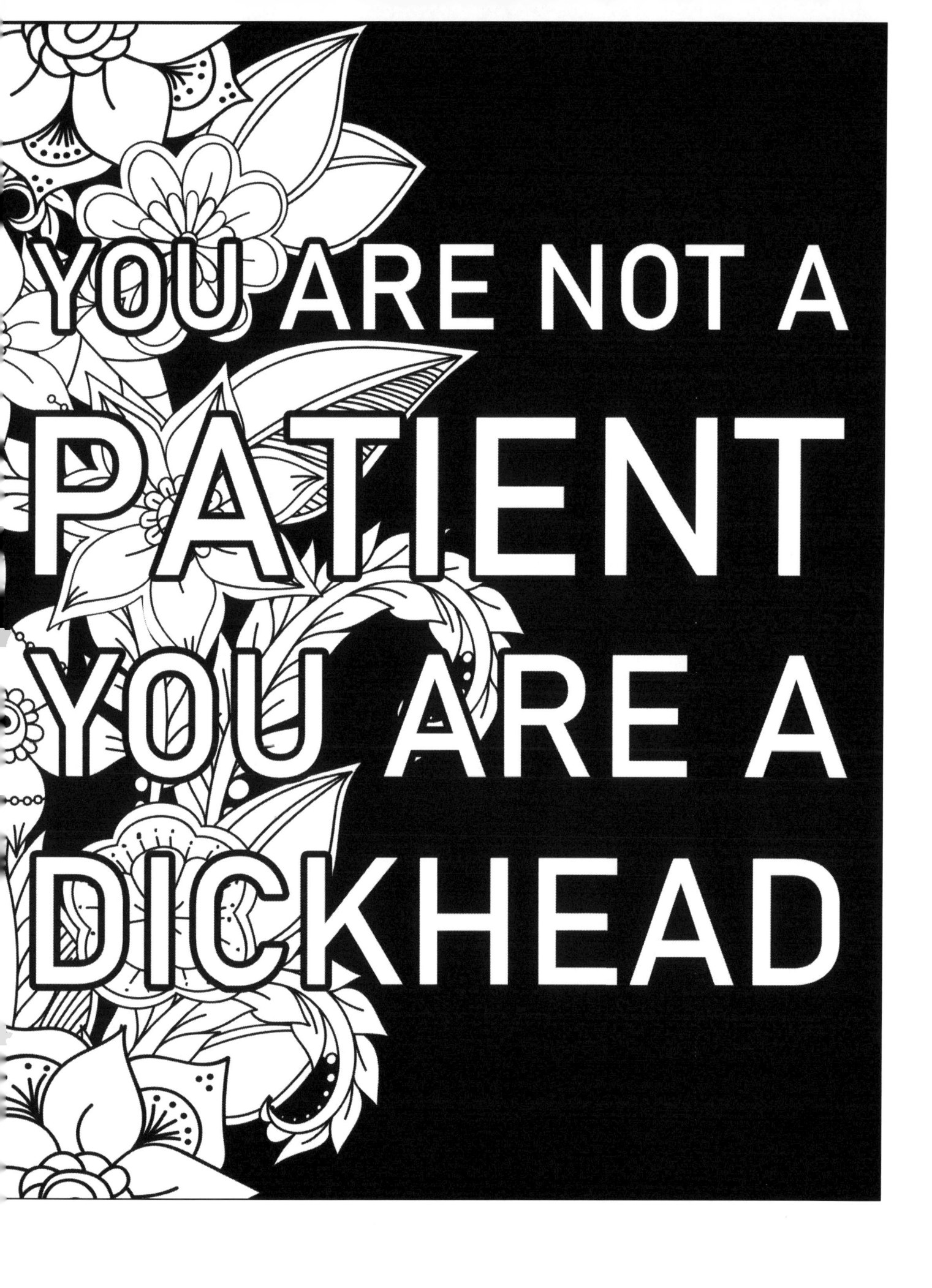

YOU ARE NOT A PATIENT YOU ARE A DICKHEAD

WEAR YOUR
FUCKING MASK

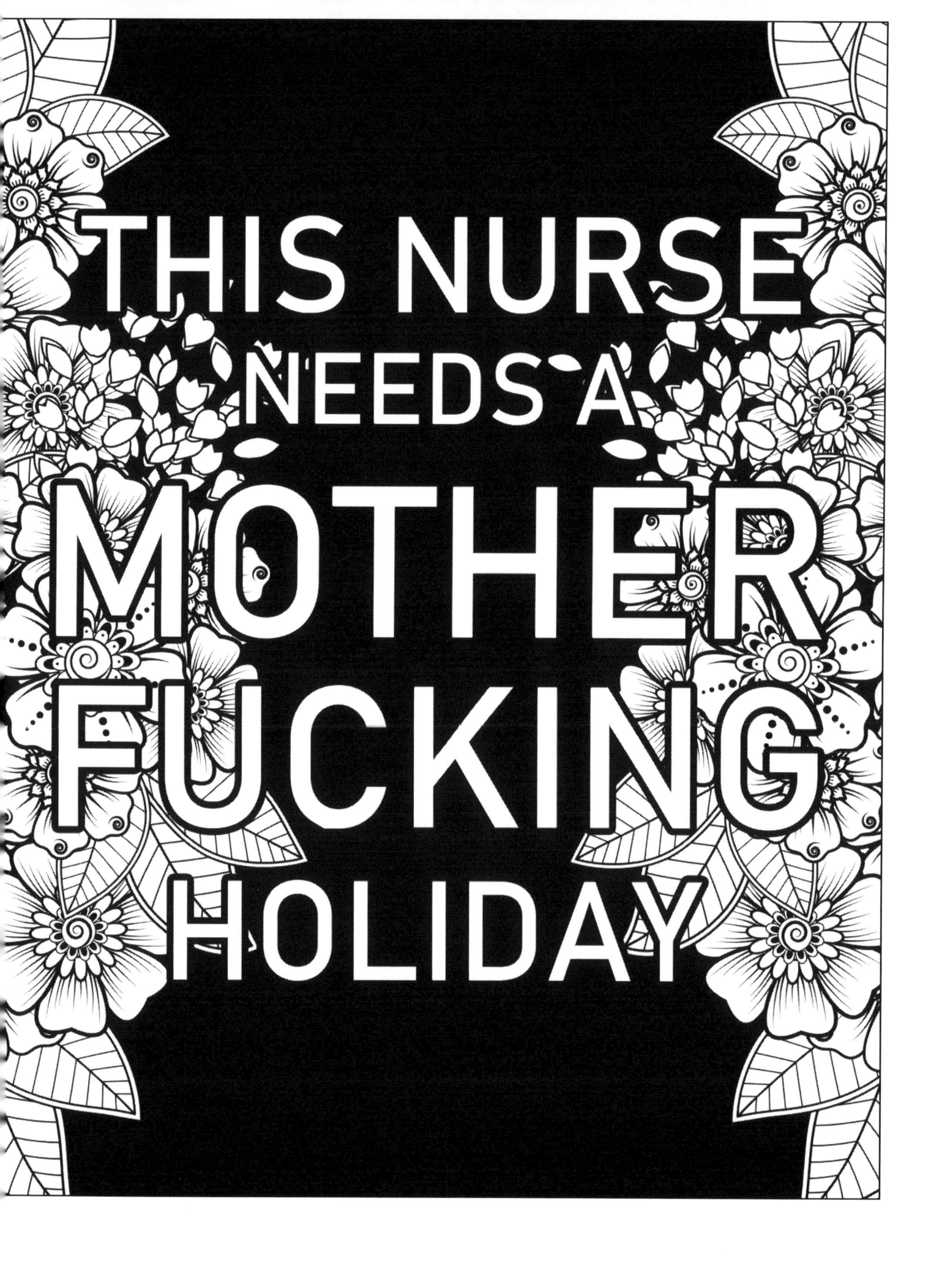

THIS NURSE NEEDS A MOTHER FUCKING HOLIDAY

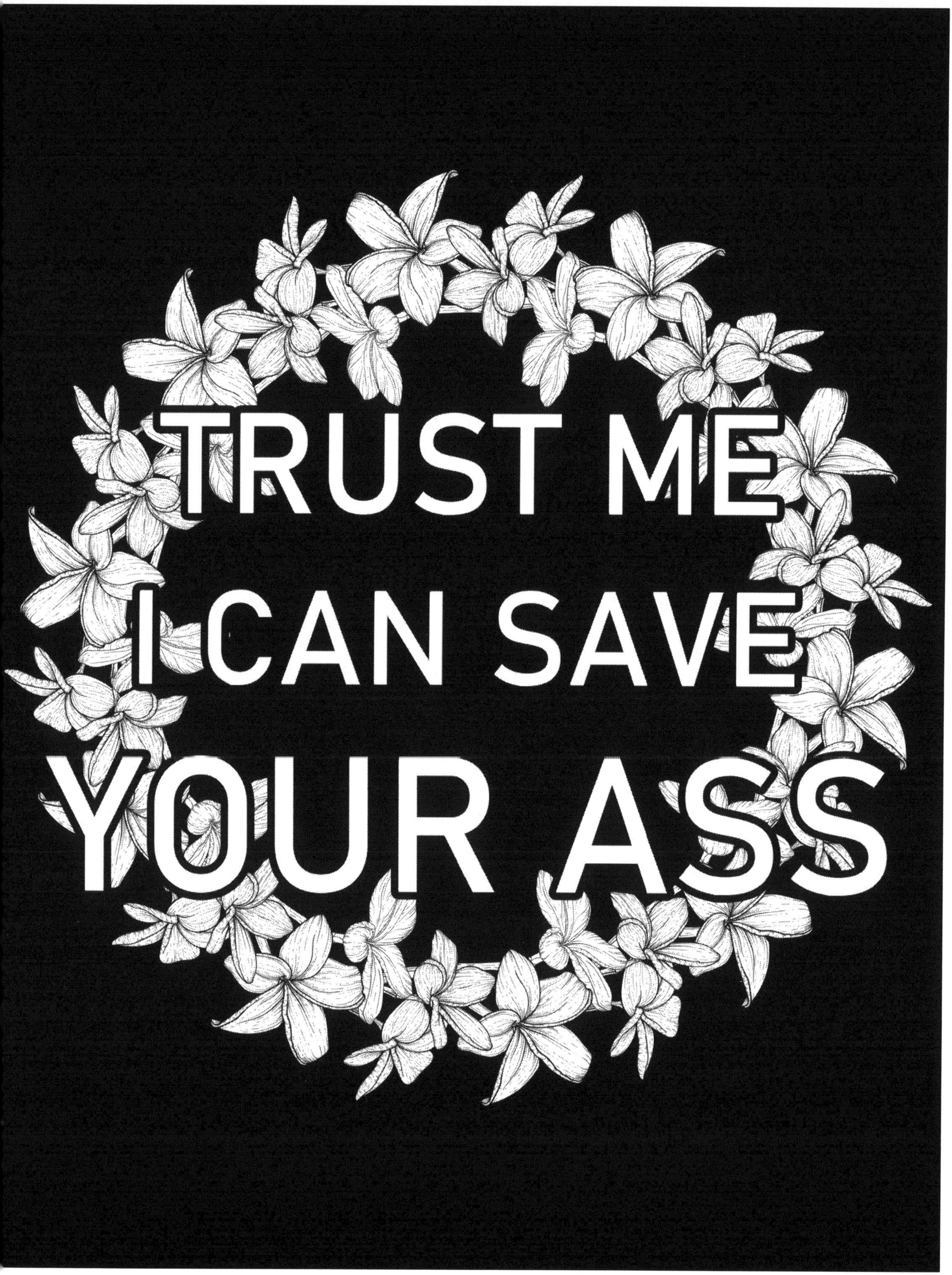
TRUST ME
I CAN SAVE
YOUR ASS

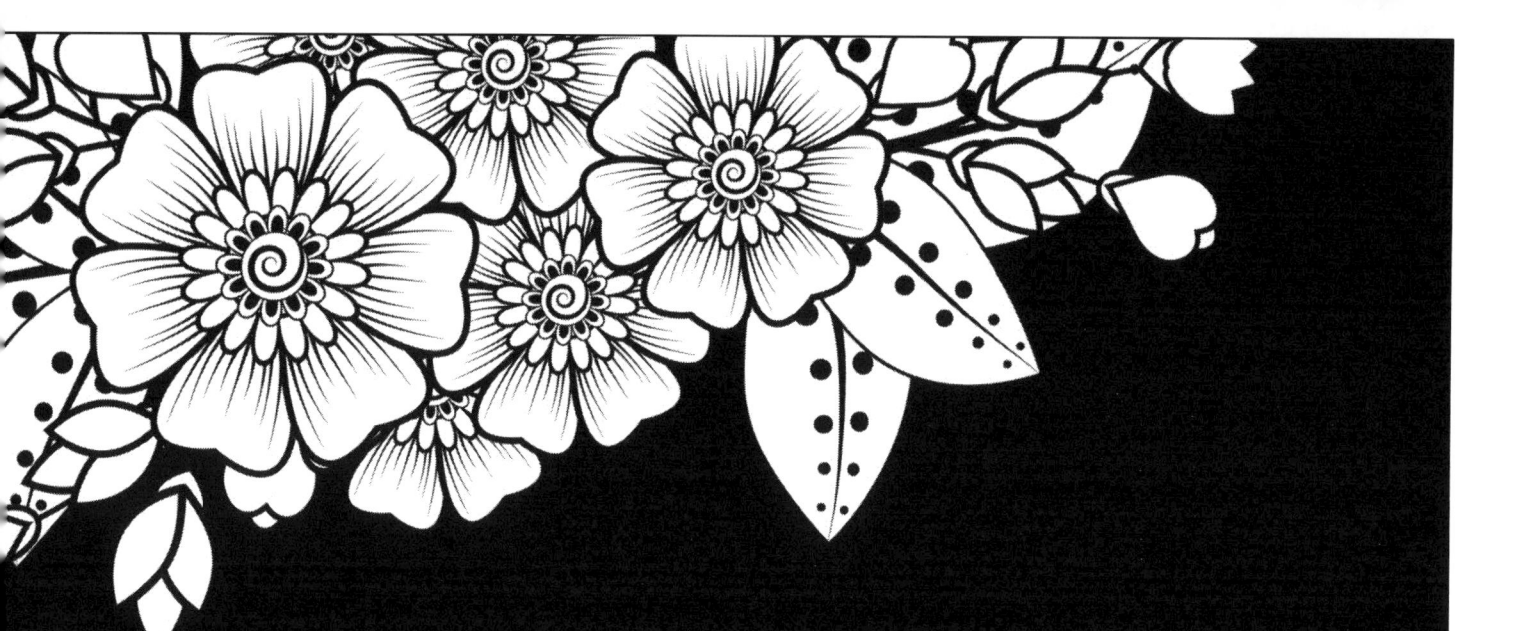

PISS OFF!
IT MY NAP TIME

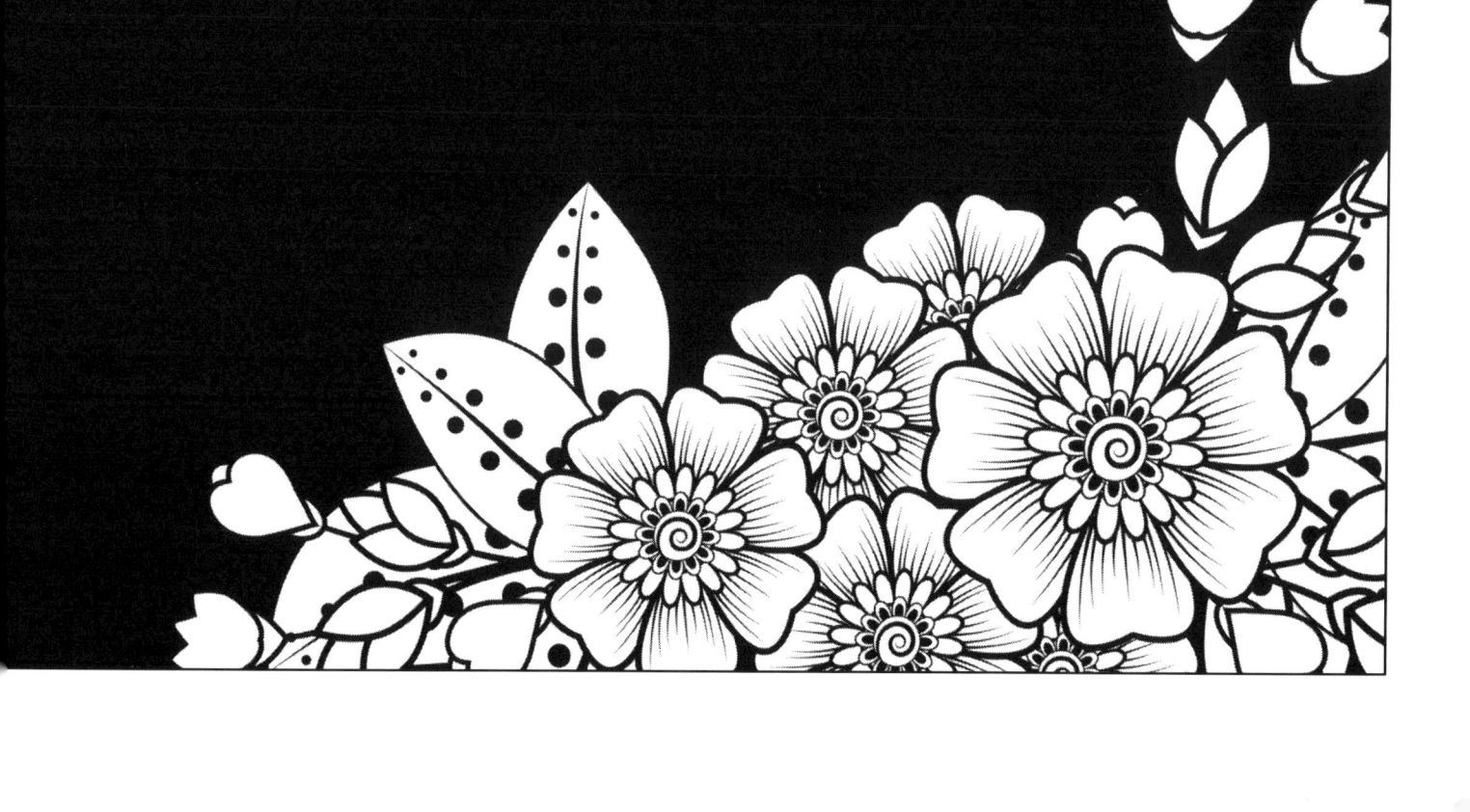

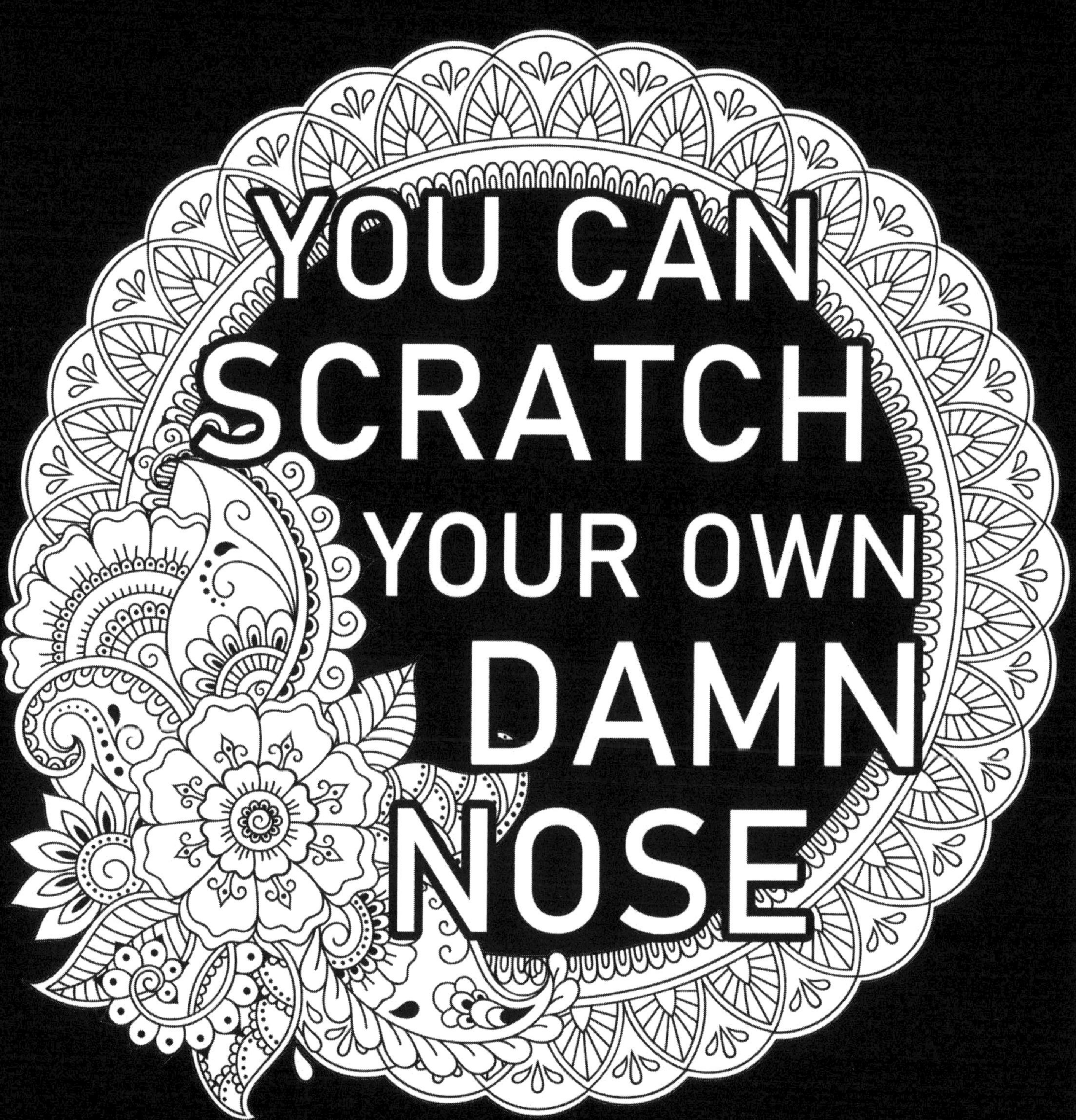
YOU CAN
SCRATCH
YOUR OWN
DAMN
NOSE

Printed in Great Britain
by Amazon